The Plant-Based Diet Starter Guide:

How to Cook, Shop, and Eat Well

Holly Yzquierdo

CONTENTS

Chapter One   1

Introduction

    My Story   1

    Can This Work for You   2

Chapter Two   3

What is a Whole Food, Plant-Based Diet

    What to Eat   3

    Foods to Avoid   6

Chapter Three   8

Getting Started

    Grocery Shopping and Reading Labels   8

    Is a Plant-Based Diet Expensive   10

    Progress Not Perfection   12

    Basic Staples   13

Chapter Four   16

Meal Planning

    Sale Price Approach   16

Chapter Five   19

Cooking for Health

    Legumes/Beans   19

    Whole Grains   20

    Cooking Veggies   20

    Baking   21

Chapter Six   24

Transitioning the Family

    Make Small Changes   24

    Go Easy on Yourself   25

    Don't Give Up   25

    Dealing with Unhappy Family   26
    Members

    My Kids Won't Eat That!   27

Chapter Seven   30

To Eat or Not to Eat

    Faux Food   30

    Smoothies & Juicing   31

    Potatoes   32

Gluten   33

Oils   33

Dairy & Eggs   35

Chapter Eight   37

But What About … A Few FAQ's

Whole Foods   37

I Feel Horrible   37

How Will I Get Enough Protein   38

Supplements   39

Nutritional Yeast   39

Chapter Nine   40

Finding the Best Approach for You

What Kind of Person Are You   40

Chapter Ten   42

Recipes

Crock Pot Mexican Rice and Bean   42
Casserole

Enchilada Soup   44

Quinoa-Lentil Tacos   45

Mexican Rice   46

Slow Cooker Potato Soup   47

Very Vegan Chili (Texas Style)   48

Basic Stir-Fry   49

Banana Bread   50

Blueberry Muffins   51

Brownies (Gluten-Free)   52

Chocolate No-Bake Bites   53

Chapter Eleven   54

Resources

About the Author   56

Chapter One

Introduction

My Story

In 2011 I was 30 years old, had recently given birth to my second child, and I was sick. The main culprit seemed to be Interstitial Cystitis (IC), an inflammatory bladder condition, also known as Painful Bladder Syndrome. IC is characterized by frequent urination, along with severe pain and discomfort—symptoms similar to a Urinary Tract Infection. Additionally, I was having uncontrollable bladder spasms. The symptoms were so severe that some days I struggled to take care of my children. Due to this condition, I was unable to leave the house without my husband's help and I had constant anxiety. I was desperate and reached out to my closest friends for help. One friend connected me with her mother, Eileen Kopsaftis, a whole food educator. Together, Eileen and I discussed my health history and current symptoms. She told me that I could be symptom-free in three months if I followed her recommendations and adopted a whole food, plant-based diet.

I committed to this new lifestyle wholeheartedly. Although there were a few bumps those first few months, I became symptom free just as Eileen had predicted! Not only that, but a couple of other unexpected things happened: I lost weight and the all-over body aches, which I had been experiencing for quite some time, disappeared! I felt (and looked) like a new person!

My husband also adopted this new lifestyle. He lost over 50 pounds and no longer needs medication for high blood pressure, high cholesterol, acid reflux, or asthma. He also stopped snoring! Isn't that extraordinary?

Can This Work for You

If you are reading this book, chances are you may have the same physical ailments which my husband and I had, or maybe you watched a thought-provoking documentary such as *Forks Over Knives*. Whatever the case, you have become convinced that the plant-based diet is the way to go, but aren't sure how to get started. My Friend, you have come to the right place. This book will explore not only what to eat, but how to shop, what and how to cook, plus offer insights to assist you to help get your family involved.

The good news is that for many unhealthy meals that you or your family eats, there is likely a healthy variation that you will come to enjoy just as much. Please know that it will take commitment. Small dietary changes can result in minor changes in your body and health for a while. If you commit to a whole food, plant-based diet for just 30 days, I believe you will feel great and get closer to a healthy weight. However, if you continue on this path beyond 30 days you will change your life.

Can you imagine growing old and feeling great? Having the energy to play with your children and grandchildren? Many people who adopt a plant-based lifestyle report achieving a healthy weight, eliminating symptoms, and reversing disease. Making positive changes now can impact your family for generations to come!

Chapter Two

What is a Whole Food, Plant-Based Diet

The whole food, plant-based diet is so much more than a diet or what you eat. It becomes a lifestyle, which can be maintained for optimal health for a lifetime.

This lifestyle focuses primarily on eating plants and whole food products, but excludes animal products such as meat and dairy and heavily refined foods such as oil. A plant-based lifestyle consists mainly of leafy greens, legumes, whole grains, vegetables, and fruits. Some people include small amounts of seeds and nuts as well. Many people who begin a plant-based lifestyle are amazed at the variety of foods available that they had never eaten before, and are equally impressed with how delicious they are.

What to Eat

As you remove things from your diet, like mentioned above, you will be adding a lot of new foods to your culinary repertoire.

Leafy Greens

I am not a salad lover by nature; believe me, it has been a process. Sometimes I eat leafy greens solely because I know that they are good for me and for my health. I need them, but it is rare that I crave leafy greens. I also don't enjoy paying bills, but I know that twice a month, without fail, it is a wise decision that serves my family well. Over time I have come to enjoy a greater variety of greens, and prefer spinach to lighter lettuces like iceberg and romaine. A large, and I'm talking serving bowl-sized large, salad is a wise idea. In addition to leafy greens, fill it with colorful veggies and fruits; include legumes and an oil-free salad dressing for a more satisfying meal.

Legumes

If the word legume (pronounced le′ gyoom) is foreign to you, think beans, peas, and lentils. Consider this a staple to be eaten every day. Legumes are typically inexpensive, especially if you purchase them dried and in bulk. Most grocery stores carry a wide variety of legumes.

Legumes are a good source of protein; they are complex carbohydrates, low in fat, and full of vitamins and naturally occurring chemical compounds called phytochemicals. They are also an excellent source of fiber, which will keep you feeling fuller longer.

Prepared Legumes can be enjoyed whole or pureed and can quickly be added to complement or substitute a variety of foods. I substitute lentils for ground beef and chickpeas for chicken all the time. Check out more ideas in the recipe section.

Whole Grains

Grains that are intact, still containing the bran, germ, and endosperm, contain all of the original nutrients and are considered *whole grains*. Whole wheat bread shouldn't be confused with whole grain bread. Some examples of whole grains include oats, brown or wild rice, wheat, quinoa (pronounced keen-wah), amaranth, millet, barley, corn, and rye. Choose those that are minimally processed (e.g., rolled, cracked, or crushed).

Don't be afraid of grains. They give you much needed fuel and fiber.

Vegetables

These are probably more familiar to you when you think of plant-based foods. Yes, broccoli, carrots, potatoes, and onions are all vegetables (but if you look in the produce aisle at your local grocery store, there are many more). Some veggies can be eaten raw, but many are enjoyed better when cooked. Many people falsely believe that potatoes are unhealthy; they can be a delicious part of the plant-based diet as they are filling and low in calories when baked. French fries, and any other fried vegetable, are not a healthy food!

Fruits

Apples, bananas, pineapples, grapes, melons, peaches, berries, and even tomatoes fall into the fruit family. Of course, there are many other fruits that I didn't mention, but these are most common in my home. Don't be afraid of the sugar found in fruit—it also contains fiber, vitamins, and phytochemicals.

Fats

I'm not referring to fried food or processed junk food. Some plants are also high in fat. A few examples include nuts, seeds, avocados, and olives. For many, these foods are not a problem, but if you are trying to reverse disease or lose a significant amount of weight, then you should avoid high-fat plant-foods.

Foods to Avoid

Animal Products

Some people who transition to a plant-based diet will still eat some animal products. If you choose to do so, I recommend that you limit them substantially. When my family and I first began our plant-based diet, we still ate meat but reduced our consumption to two to three ounces (usually beef or chicken) only two or three times per week. We also limited our consumption of eggs and completely eliminated dairy.

If you are hoping to reverse or eliminate disease, I encourage you to eliminate all animal products. There will be people who tell you this isn't healthy, but hang in there.

Oil

We also eliminated oil. Oil is pure fat. It has zero nutrients, unlike its plant counterparts which will be discussed later in the book. If you eat olives you will consume fat, but also fiber and nutrients.

Highly Processed Food

Most processed food is junk and should not be consumed *regularly*. Later, I'll give you some guidelines to help you determine what junk should be eliminated completely.

But I Can't Live Without...

If you think you can't live without animal products, but really want to try to eat a plant-based diet, then start slowly. Perhaps you could schedule certain days that you will eat small amounts of animal products. For example, you may choose to eat meat on Friday nights when you go out, or have ice cream on Sundays. I'm not saying you can never have these things again, but I encourage you to really give it a try. Remember, this is a lifestyle change, and, therefore, it is a process. I discovered a healthy baseline after adopting a plant-based diet. I could occasionally eat meat without adverse effects (digestive trouble), but dairy was a big no-no for me. It caused severe pain and inflammation so I chose not to eat dairy.

Eventually we decided that we wouldn't eat any animal-based products at home; we would reserve them for eating out. I'll still have a salad dressing with oil occasionally, but only at a restaurant. This worked well for us since we ate out often enough and didn't feel deprived. Soon I made the decision to abstain from meat even when eating out.

Chapter Three

Getting Started

Before you can eat healthy you will need to learn how to buy and store healthy food.

Grocery Shopping and Reading Labels

Once you make the transition to a whole food, plant-based diet you may find that much of the food you eat will not have a nutrition label. Produce doesn't normally have a label unless it is in a prepackaged container. Foods that come in containers, like berries, mushrooms, and salads, will have a label. Often, foods that can be bought in bulk bins, like beans and grains, may have nutrition labels near the bin, but isn't necessarily on the food you purchase and take home. The following guidelines will help you understand nutrition labels. Please note that your first few shopping trips will likely take longer than usual.

Understanding Nutrition Labels

The nutrition label is the box, usually on the back or side of the product, which lists serving size, calories, fat, fiber, vitamins, etc. It is typically followed by a list of ingredients. The guidelines for nutrition labels vary by country, so I will discuss some of the general things you should look for.

I find the most important part of the nutrition label to be the ingredients section. Food manufacturers are required to disclose all ingredients used in their products. Ingredients are listed in descending order, meaning the ingredients at the top of the list make up more of the product. For example, peanut butter often says, "peanuts, sugar, oil, salt". Obviously, peanuts make up the majority of the product, but sugar could be a significant portion as well.

You may find some ingredients listed as *natural flavors* or *spices*, which make it really difficult to determine what is in the product. Many additives and chemicals fall into this legal loop hole. Personally, I feel that if a company doesn't disclose everything that is in the product, I do not want to purchase it.

Manipulating the Ingredient List

Even with safeguards in place ingredient labels can be manipulated, so it is important to understand the ingredients and their derivatives in the products you purchase. For example, many ready-to-eat cereals are full of sugar. Many people wouldn't want to buy a cereal that lists sugar as the first ingredient. Remember that the first ingredient makes up that biggest percentage of the product's content. Instead of listing sugar as the first ingredient, food companies may use various types of sugar, including corn syrup and high-fructose corn syrup. By using different forms of sweeteners, sugar may be listed as the second or third ingredient instead of the first. Therefore, sugar in its various forms could make up the bulk of your product.

I compared ingredient labels for cereals that most people would consider healthy. The first cereal lists whole grain oats, *sugar*, oat bran, modified corn starch, *honey*, and *brown sugar syrup* as the top six ingredients. This cereal's serving size is three quarters of a cup, which includes nine grams of sugar. The second cereal lists whole grain wheat, raisins, wheat bran, *sugar*, *brown sugar syrup*, and salt in its top six ingredients, recording 18 grams of sugar for a one cup serving.

You can see how it is difficult to understand exactly what and how much you are consuming.

Serving Sizes

You must also take a look at the serving sizes listed on the label. Most cereal bowls hold two cups of cereal. I would bet that most people eat at least that much when they have cereal for breakfast. In the cereal example above, a person who ate two cups of the first cereal would consume 24 grams of sugar (plus milk) and 36 grams of sugar from the second cereal.

Another example of deceptive labeling is non-stick spray oil. According to the nutrition label, spray oil contains zero calories and zero fat per serving. A serving is indicated as one quarter of a second spray. Most people will spray for several seconds. We know that oil, even spray oil, is 100% fat. However, by listing such a small serving size, the label misleads you into believing the spray is harmless.

Don't Trust the Packaging

Although the nutrition label is sometimes difficult to decipher, never trust what is on the front of the package. Companies can put any advertising they want on the package. Statements can be misleading: "Now with 50% more protein", "More Fiber", "Heart Healthy", and "Low Fat" are only a few of the buzzwords that can lead you astray. The nutrition label on the back is the only way to accurately know what is in the product.

Is a Plant-Based Diet Expensive

Some people worry that eating a plant-based diet will be too expensive, but we save money eating this way. Meat and dairy products tend to be expensive while produce, beans, grains, and potatoes are inexpensive. You can save money by buying seasonal produce and buying some ingredients in bulk.

Should I Buy Organic

There are many different opinions about organic food. Some of the food I buy is organic but much of it is not. I don't go out of my way to purchase organic food and only do when we can afford it. I have friends who purchase mostly organic food; they prioritize it in their budget, but not everyone can afford to do so.

Organic Doesn't Mean Healthy

It is easy to find organic products at most grocery stores. However, they are usually much more expensive than their conventional counterparts. Cookies, crackers, chips, muffins—you name it and there are organic versions available. The *organic* label doesn't necessarily make it healthy and shouldn't give you a license to buy it. Think about it, conventional fruit is always healthier than organic chips!

Every year the Environmental Working Group updates two lists: the Clean Fifteen and the Dirty Dozen. The Clean Fifteen is a list of produce that is less likely to be contaminated by pesticides while the Dirty Dozen consists of produce most likely to be contaminated. These lists can be a helpful guide as you choose how to allocate your grocery budget.

Food I Typically Buy Organic

- Corn Tortilla Chips (these are not a regular purchase)
- Quinoa
- Strawberries
- Sugar
- Flour (wheat and gluten-free)

Progress Not Perfection

Big changes can be overwhelming, but there is no need to transform your kitchen overnight. Yes, you will reap more benefits if you completely change your diet, but if you need to take small steps, that's OK. Small steps in the right direction are still progress. Experiment with one or two new ingredients each week as your budget allows.

Having a plan and a shopping list can significantly reduce your grocery bill whether you eat plant-based or not. I prepare weekly meal plans that serve as a guideline for our week. I don't stress about following it closely, but it helps to have a plan for the week. You can find more information on meal planning and a sample meal plan in the next chapter.

The Great Pantry Clean Out

Buying healthy food is important, but you must also get all of the unhealthy food out of your reach. This can be hard. I don't like to throw away food, even unhealthy food. When we made the switch, our freezer and pantry were both full of meat, dairy, and plenty of processed items. Non-perishable items that were not opened or expired were donated. We also gave away grocery bags filled with frozen meat, cheese, and butter. Our last hurrah came when a friend had a baby: I prepared some of the meat and pasta and made her five different meals she could eat that week or freeze for later.

I felt better about the loss of money spent on the food we would not eat, knowing it was going to help others.

It is difficult to eat healthy when your pantry is full of junk. You will reach for the foods that take the least amount of time to prepare—a quick fix. Chips and cupcakes will disappear long before cabbage and cucumbers.

Generally, you should eliminate the following pantry foods:

- Expired
- Containing ingredients that you can't pronounce or don't recognize
- Containing white flour or white sugar
- Containing high-fructose corn syrup
- Represented by a mascot (A mascot is an animated character used to sell the product.)
- Containing more than five ingredients

Exceptions to the five-ingredients rule:

- Multi-grain baking mixes
- Multi-grain breads
- Healthy Soups
- Condiments that have good (or better) ingredients

Schedule a day and time to clean out the unhealthy foods from your kitchen. Depending on the size of your pantry and the amount of food in your refrigerator and freezer, you may need to spread it out over a weekend. Once you have cleaned out your kitchen of all things bad for you, you may be wondering, "What should I buy?"

Basic Staples

Here is my list of basic ingredients I *almost* always have available.

Spices

Black/white pepper   Chili powder
Cinnamon   Garlic powder
Onion powder   Sea salt
Turmeric   Cumin

Pantry

Agave nectar   Applesauce
Baking Soda   Brown rice
Baking Powder   Vanilla
Canned beans   Whole grain cereal
Chocolate chips (non-dairy)   Cocoa
Coffee   Dried beans
Dried fruits   Flour
Grains   Shelf-stable non-dairy milks
Nutritional yeast   Nuts/seeds
Old-fashioned oats   Pasta
Pasta sauce   Quinoa
Raw sugar   Red wine vinegar
Tomato sauce   Tortillas
Tortilla chips   Turbinado sugar

Freezer

Bananas   Blueberries
Breads   Cherries
Corn   Mixed veggies
Strawberries   Whole wheat pastry flour

Refrigerator

Rice milk	Apple butter
Applesauce	Braggs Liquid Aminos
Coconut milk coffee creamer	Fat-free balsamic vinaigrette
Flax seeds	Jelly (with no added sugar)
Lemon/lime juice	Mustard
Natural nut butters	Nutritional yeast
Dates	Maple syrup
Salsa	Sunflower seed butter

Fresh Produce

Apples	Bananas
Broccoli	Carrots
Garlic	Onions
Potatoes	Sweet potatoes
Spinach and other lettuces	Peppers
Other seasonal produce	

I can make most of my recipes with these ingredients. I did not buy them all at once and I don't use them all the time, but these are my essentials. When I have people over they are usually overwhelmed by the fullness of my pantry.

Depending on your tastes and cooking style, you may have a different list of essentials. Your list could change over time, too. For example, my son has multiple food allergies that we have discovered since transitioning to a plant-based diet. I no longer buy nuts in bulk because he has nut allergies.

For an up to date list of Basic Staples visit
http://myplantbasedfamily.com/basic-staples/

Chapter Four

Meal Planning

There are two approaches to meal planning which I utilize: sale price and family favorites. Either can work well, but both require a little planning before you go to the store. The longer you plan, the easier it gets.

Sale Price Approach

Most grocery stores send out weekly circulars featuring sale items for that week. This usually includes a fair amount of items that are marked down a significant amount below their normal retail price called *loss leaders*. I have always been a loss leader shopper to some degree. For example, maybe apples are normally $0.99 per pound, but this week they are $0.50 per pound. That is a loss leader.

To use this approach, take out a notebook and write all of the loss leaders you are even remotely interested in for the store you are shopping. If you have a store that ad matches, you can write the loss leaders for every store in which you have a circular. Then you start matching items to meals.

Another benefit to doing this system for a while is that you figure out how much food generally costs so you know when there is a good deal and you can stock up on those items in your pantry. This system is also particularly helpful for budget-conscious people.

Family Favorite Rotation Approach

This approach doesn't necessarily check ad prices, but it does take seasonal produce (which is generally less expensive) into account. Your rotation could be weekly, bi-weekly, monthly, or even every six weeks. I recommend starting out with a weekly or bi-weekly plan to give you more flexibility.

When using this approach, make a list of your family's favorite recipes and the ingredients you need for each. If you keep a well-stocked pantry you may not need to buy all of the items. For example, I always have a variety of beans and grains in my pantry so my shopping list would not include these items, but I would need to make note of the fresh veggies needed.

Some families enjoy theme nights: Taco Tuesday, Pasta Wednesday, Pizza Friday, etc. My kids always like the predictability of having their favorites regularly. Once or twice a week have a new recipe night so you can try new things and phase out some of the meals that have worn out their welcome.

Sample Meal Plan

Day One
Breakfast: Blueberry oatmeal
Lunch: Veggie wrap
Dinner: Nachos or tostadas

Day Two
Breakfast: Breakfast quinoa
Lunch: Baked potato and salad
Dinner: Veggie pasta and side salad

Day Three
Breakfast: Whole grain toast with nut butter and fresh fruit
Lunch: Bean and rice burrito
Dinner: Chili and baked potato wedges

Day Four
Breakfast: Whole grain cereal with fruit
Lunch: Bean and grain bowl
Dinner: Portobello steaks, dirty mashed potatoes, and steamed broccoli

Day Five
Breakfast: Apple cinnamon oatmeal
Lunch: Taco salad
Dinner: Lentil shepherd's pie

Chapter Five

Cooking for Health

Our diet includes beans, grains, cooked and raw veggies, and fruit, along with some baked goods. This section will give you a quick guide to cooking these foods.

Legumes/Beans

Most legumes take a long time to cook if you buy them dried. Dried beans are less expensive than canned beans and are also free of additives.

How to Cook Dry Beans

First, sort the dry beans, removing any sticks, rocks, or debris, and rinse well. I use a colander.

Second, soak the beans overnight, leaving plenty of room for the beans to double in size. I usually fill my pot half way with beans and all of the way with water.

Third, the next day rinse the beans again and add fresh water.

Last, cook over medium heat until beans are soft. One small tip: If you take a few beans into a spoon and gently blow on them, the skins will split and slowly peel when they are done. The cooking time will vary by bean type.

Spices and vegetables can be added to the beans while they are cooking. I'll often cook pinto beans with a dry bay leaf, half an onion, and a few cloves of garlic. Occasionally, I'll add some hot peppers to increase the spiciness and add a unique flavor.

Some legumes, like lentils, are quick-cooking and cook more like grains. For lentils, simply rinse well then add one part lentil and two parts water; cook on medium heat until done (about 20 minutes).

Whole Grains

Cooking techniques and cooking times vary depending on the type of grain, but many grains, such as rice, barley, bulgur, amaranth, wheat groats, and quinoa, can be cooked by rinsing well and then following the one part grain, two parts water rule. Some recipes will require more water (or other liquid). Grains usually do best when covered with a lid to avoid water loss. If the grains are done but water remains, simply uncover and cook for a few more minutes. I allow more liquid when I'm making oatmeal, soups, stews, or casseroles.

Cooking Veggies

Steaming

Many vegetables and fruits can be steamed by placing them in a steamer basket over boiling water with a lid. Hard vegetables, like carrots, will take longer than softer veggies, like asparagus or broccoli. Although I'm not a big fan of the microwave, many people use them and they can help busy families get a hot meal on the table quickly. Some companies sell vegetable side dishes in steamer bags, where you just put the whole bag in the microwave for a specific amount of time. You can also purchase empty steamer bags to use with fresh produce. Our microwave has a *steam* button as well. If you are anti-microwave I understand your complaint, but I think vegetables cooked in the microwave are still better than drive-thru cheeseburgers.

Sautéing

Sautéing is my favorite method for cooking vegetables because it is so quick and easy. Although you are not technically *frying* anything, you can still enjoy an amazing meal without the oil. If you have traditionally cooked with a lot of oil, you may feel a little lost as you transition away from it. Believe me, as your taste buds change (and they will), you will develop a new appreciation for the way food tastes.

Water or veggie broth make a zero calorie oil substitution that will leave your veggies clean and crisp. I begin most stir-fries with onions, peppers, and sometimes mushrooms: these three veggies will render their own juices as they cook. If they begin to stick, I add small amounts of water or broth to the pan— not oil. Then I add other, harder veggies, such as broccoli and/or carrots. Finally, I add cooked grains and/or beans, and sometimes fruit. These tend to stick to everything as soon as they hit the pan, so use low heat.

Roasting

I have friends who love to roast veggies, but think it must be done with oil. This is not true. Simply wash and cut veggies the way you normally would, then place them into a shallow, oven-safe pan. Fresh herbs, spices, and veggie broth can be sprinkled on the veggies, then roast as the recipe indicates. You may need to stir the veggies occasionally to help them cook evenly.

Baking

Transitioning to a plant-based lifestyle does not mean you have to give up baking. In fact, you can still enjoy your family favorites by substituting the top three worst offenders: **dairy, oil, and white sugar**.

Replacing Dairy

Dairy is usually added to baked goods in the form of milk, butter, and yogurt. Milk is easy to replace: simply substitute your favorite non-dairy milk. I prefer to use rice milk when I bake because it has a very mild flavor and, if my family ends up sharing treats, I don't have to worry about allergies. Butter can be replaced by adding mashed banana or applesauce; I usually avoid vegan butters because they are high in fat and low in nutrients. Dairy yogurt can be replaced with non-dairy yogurt.

Replacing Oil

I often replace oil or butter with applesauce or mashed bananas, but pureed prunes are also a great option. Since applesauce and mashed bananas are both used as my top replacements for butter or oil (and also eggs) in a recipe, I am careful to not use more than one cup of either because it can change the constitution of the baked item.

I've mentioned that you don't need to add oil to baked goods, but you may be wondering how to keep them from sticking to the pan. There are a few options: when making muffins you can use baking cups (some are specially designed to keep muffins from sticking); you could invest in silicone bakeware; and parchment paper is a great non-stick option that makes clean up a breeze.

Confession: To make it easier, I use non-stick cooking spray (oil) when cooking pancakes. I usually only spray it once at the beginning of cooking so it adds minimal fat.

Replacing White Sugar

There are many options to replace white sugar. I usually reduce the sugar by half for most recipes. I'll also replace white sugar with maple syrup, date paste, or turbinado sugar. Choosing healthier recipes helps, too. For example, one of my muffin recipes calls for a half cup of sugar for 12 muffins, which is about two tsp. of sugar per muffin. Most muffin recipes call for at least one cup of sugar, sometimes more. Since I replace oil and dairy with fruit most of the time, which add sweetness to the recipe, larger amounts of sugar are not necessary.

Chapter Six

Transitioning the Family

I get a lot of emails from readers who have watched *Forks Over Knives* or read a book about reversing disease, and they are ready to change their diet to get healthy. For many, the idea of completely changing their diet seems overwhelming and impossible. Even if you commit to this lifestyle you'll likely have family members who do not share in your commitment. Please know that while it may be difficult, it is possible and totally worth it!

The most difficult situation seems to arise when one spouse wants to change and the other does not. Many families end up making multiple meals to please everyone in the family. I would have had a hard time sticking with it if I had to make a meal for me, a different one for my husband, and still a separate meal for our kids! So I design most of my recipes to easily incorporate meat, but it isn't the main event.

The following tips will help you as you transition your family to a whole food, plant-based diet.

Make Small Changes

No one says you have to give up meat, dairy, or eggs overnight. Initially, we cut back to two to three ounces of meat two or three times per week. We didn't feel deprived; in fact, we felt great. I would buy meat at the store, then, as soon as I got home, I would cut the meat into small portions and freeze them. Eventually, I was only buying meat for my husband and would cook it separately in a small pan.

After a few months, I was pretty grossed out at the thought of meat and didn't want to cook it anymore. If we ate meat it was on our regular date night. Most of the time only my husband would order meat and I would order a vegan meal.

Go Easy on Yourself

Unlike other decisions, choosing to eat plant-based isn't a make-it-or-break-it thing. Sure, a plant-based diet has been shown to prevent and reverse disease, but if you give in and buy a cheeseburger, the walls are not going to come crumbling down. Maybe you will even give yourself permission to eat a steak once a month or indulge in some other favorite. Go ahead. If that makes it easier for you to eat healthy, do it. After a while, you may decide you don't need or want that appointment with yourself. You may lose a taste for your (former) favorite meal, or feel ill after you have it.

Don't Give Up

Sometimes I find myself in a slump. I don't really feel like cooking or shopping for food. I just want to sit and eat whatever is quick and easiest. There have been times where we practically lived on take-out bean burritos! Yes, they may be better than cheeseburgers but they are still full of additives, oils, and who knows what! So, do you want to know what I do? I just keep going. I don't give up because I had a bad day, week, or month (yes month). I just keep going. I do my best to get back on track. I don't keep my eyes on an unattainable idea of perfection. The way I eat IS NOT PERFECT, but it is much better than it was when I ate the Standard American Diet (SAD).

Dealing with Unhappy Family Members

I feel it is very important to honor your spouse. If you are interested in eating a plant-based diet and your spouse is not, please don't use my guidelines to create a rift between the two of you. Honor and serve one another. If my husband really wanted me to cook meat for him, I would. I would not wreck our relationship over food.

This can be applied to relationships with children, friends, and extended family. Our kids don't dictate what they eat mainly because they are young. They do have some input and frequently make requests. However, when our older children visit from out of state, I try to honor their dietary choices without compromising ours. I will create a menu with healthy plant-based foods, some of their old unhealthy favorites, and choose some restaurants with a good selection of food for all of us. If they lived with us all the time, we would come up with a different plan. The key is communicating healthy and respectful boundaries.

I often hear of horrible stories of extended family members going behind the parents' backs to give kids junk food. I think the response will vary with each individual situation, and there is no right answer. I do my best to make sure anyone with my kids understands what they can and cannot have, and explain the reasons why. I usually pack all of their food for such outings, and save special treats for these occasions. I wouldn't leave my kids with someone unless I trust them to follow my rules.

My friendships have changed somewhat, too. Many people think I eat only super healthy, home-grown, organic, weird food. Therefore, I don't get invited to many parties or events. When I do, I always offer to bring something and try to wow everyone with how good plant-based fare can taste. I have come to accept the fact that for some, my (perceived) food choices make them uncomfortable, or maybe even intimidated. I try to be casual about it, not wanting to shove it down anyone's throat. Many times it seems it is all we can talk about. The good news, though, is sometimes I get calls and texts from friends who have decided to take the plunge into a healthier way of eating, and I get to be their tour guide.

My Kids Won't Eat That! Tips to Get Your Kids Eating Healthy

Kids and food—it will always be a struggle, whether you eat plant-based or SAD. Different families have different dynamics, so rules that work for one family will not always work for another. Instead of offering rules though, I have some tips that will help kids (or spouses) adjust to new foods.

Be a Good Example

If you want your kids to eat healthy, then you must eat healthy. They don't understand why there are different rules about food for kids and grownups. Our kids ALWAYS want what we're eating. Every Saturday morning, my husband will make a giant bowl of spinach with blueberries, broccoli, red bell peppers, and any other fruit we may have. Our kids devour this meal; they want to eat what their dad eats.

Use a Dip

My kids, dare I say all kids, love to eat foods they can dip. Whether it is ketchup (don't forget to read the label), salad dressing, peanut butter, barbeque sauce, or marinara, kids love to dip their food—even more so if it is in a fun bowl. Raw spinach leaves in my blueberry salad dressing and sliced red bell peppers in hummus are personal favorites of theirs.

Clever Combinations

The dip tip mentioned above goes hand in hand with clever combinations. Simply adding cinnamon to a dish will often win over a picky eater. If your kid won't eat beans, puree them and add them to a tostada or give them chips to scoop up the beans. That combination is a winner with kids and a hesitant spouse. Maybe they won't eat quinoa, so try adding fresh berries and making it into a breakfast or dessert with a drizzle of maple syrup. The possibilities are endless.

Offer New Foods Often

It may take many tries to get your kids to accept new foods. I offered my boys dried seaweed (I know it sounds weird), but it took several attempts for my kids to accept it. Now they ask for it.

Abstain If Necessary

When we discovered our son had extensive nut allergies, I traded in our peanut and almond butters and made the switch to sunflower seed butter. Our boys did not want to eat sunflower seed butter sandwiches—they would refuse to eat lunch. I decided to avoid sandwiches for about a month. Then I reintroduced the sunflower seed butter and something magical happened: they loved sunflower seed butter sandwiches! They would eat them every day if I let them!

Make Exceptions

If your child can understand, "we don't eat this every day, this is a sometimes food", then I don't see harm in allowing kids to eat food that would normally be off limits. Let me try to explain. We attended a friend's birthday party where our four year old was allowed to have a cupcake, complete with a tower of frosting on top. However, our two year old, with multiple food allergies, was not. He understands (he is very wise) that sometimes we eat fries, but he knows that he cannot eat wheat, dairy, peanuts, and the list goes on. Some kids may not handle sometimes situations well. Our kids are thrilled when they are allowed sometimes food, and, yes, they ask for it and they get disappointed when they can't have something they request. As children learn more about healthy and unhealthy foods, it will be easier to handle social situations. Talking about what they may encounter, and why you do or do not eat certain foods, will help as well.

Chapter Seven

To Eat or Not to Eat

If you've paid any attention over the last decade to what the media claims is healthy, you may be really confused. The general public is completely confused about what constitutes good nutrition. Medical experts don't always help this confusion; they are often completely for or against certain foods, without regard for an individual's specific medical needs.

Remember, I am not a doctor and this doesn't constitute medical advice; this is just my common-sense approach to navigating the dos and don'ts of healthy eating. Now I'll discuss faux foods, smoothies, potatoes, gluten, oil/fat, and dairy.

Faux Food

As soon as people decide to remove meat from their diet they start looking for an alternative. Unfortunately, most meat alternatives you'll find are unhealthy, food-like products that I call faux food. Faux foods, sometimes called fake foods, often contain questionable ingredients or involve some nutrient-robbing processes that counteract the original benefits. These types of foods are not a healthy replacement for real, whole food. I think faux foods can be an acceptable part of a plant-based diet if they are used occasionally. By occasionally, I mean holidays or special occasions. You should still be very careful and read the ingredients, because many faux products still contain ingredients that I feel are unacceptable. One such ingredient is casein. Casein comes from milk and is in many faux meat and faux cheese products. If you watched *Forks Over Knives*, you may recall that Dr. Campbell fed rats the animal-protein casein and a carcinogen, and the rats developed cancer. Rats that were fed the carcinogen and plant-protein did not develop cancer.

I have seen faux lunch meat and cheese products that contain really scary ingredients. Products like that should not be a regular part of a healthy, plant-based diet.

Other products, like rice and almond milk, may be considered faux milk, but many use very clean ingredients and are acceptable as a daily part of this lifestyle. I still encourage you to read the label before buying any products.

Smoothies & Juicing

There are two main camps: one is in favor of juicing and smoothies and the other is strongly opposed. I'll give you a brief summary of each stance, fill you in on my opinion, and let you choose for yourself.

Those in favor of juicing and smoothies stress all of the vitamins, antioxidants, and good nutrition that someone gets from juicing or blending a wide variety of veggies and fruits. It would be hard for me to consume a bunch of kale, half a dozen carrots and celery, and a few pounds of apples, but if those are juiced or blended it would be much easier. I know a lot of people who have seen positive changes in their health through juicing and smoothies.

Those against juicing and smoothies say that it is better to consume the whole food. By eating the whole food you get all of the fiber, since it isn't removed as pulp or blended up, losing some of its properties. Additionally, they say it isn't natural to drink juices or smoothies, as those that do consume more calories than necessary, without the much needed fiber to balance it out.

I understand both camps and I don't typically drink juices or smoothies. For me, I'd rather have the whole food—it's really more of a taste and texture preference. My husband and sons love juices and smoothies, and would have them every day if I would make them. Unfortunately for them, I don't like to clean the blender or juicer. I also find it costs more. When I make smoothies, I use lots of spinach, bananas, berries, oranges, and rice milk: the cost for those ingredients can add up. I find it cheaper to eat the fruit; I get full before I finish it.

You can pick either camp. Your personal preference, dietary requirements, and budget situation will be contributing factors. If you have kids (or a spouse) that won't eat veggies, then try a smoothie. If they love eating raw veggies, then stick with that. Just remember, if you are trying to decide if smoothies or juicing is the best for you and your family, then you are probably not eating the Standard American Diet. More than likely you are making healthy decisions for your family.

Potatoes

I had a reader email me saying she had not eaten potatoes in 15 years. I couldn't believe it. She wanted to be healthy and had heard that carbs were bad, so she avoided starchy vegetables in an effort to lose weight and get healthy.

The problem with that is potatoes are a low calorie food that do a great job of filling us up and providing us with energy. I challenge you to replace one form of processed food, such as bread, granola bars, or cookies, with a baked potato, and see if it makes a difference. Remember, it isn't the potato that's bad, but what you put on it.

Gluten

I'm sure you've seen "gluten-free" labels in the grocery store. If you aren't familiar with gluten, it is a protein found in barley, rye, and wheat. Oats are usually cross-contaminated because they are processed on shared equipment. Some people have jumped on the gluten-free bandwagon as a way to lose weight. That could work. If you typically eat a lot of breads, pastas, or other products that are gluten-heavy, eliminating them could help you lose weight. Those products are often heavily processed. Elimination of highly processed food of any kind will help with weight loss.

There is a growing population of gluten-intolerant and gluten-sensitive people in the United States. Many people note digestive issues with symptoms ranging from diarrhea to constipation. Other symptoms can include skin problems, hair loss, ADD, fatigue, headaches, nausea, joint pain, and the list goes on. Do a quick search on Google and you will be amazed by what you find. Some people also have allergies to gluten and develop a condition called celiac disease, in which the lining of the small intestine is damaged and nutrients are prevented from being absorbed. However, if you don't have any problems with grains containing gluten, they can be an incredibly healthy and filling part of your diet.

Many people tell me they experience a relief of symptoms within days of going gluten-free, and lose several pounds within the first week. However, it is important to note that it takes a long time for gluten to get out of your system, and it must be completely eliminated to evaluate its effect on you.

Oils

The media has bombarded us with the idea that we need oil to be healthy. I was never a big fan of oil, and would try to leave it out when I could. I remember seeing olive oil in the supermarket and buying it because it claimed to be good for my heart. Headlines claim olive oil is "heart healthy" and fish have "good fat". I recently watched a documentary claiming cholesterol was good for us, not differentiating between HDL, good cholesterol, and LDL, bad cholesterol.

Yes, our bodies need fat to survive, but we don't need added oil to be healthy. I have many friends on the olive oil and coconut oil bandwagon; I was once there as well. People with active lifestyles, who eat a healthy diet, may not experience health problems related to oil consumption, but I have not found that to be the norm.

Individuals with medical conditions are better off limiting any added fat.

How to Eat Fat

We can get all of the fat we need from plants: nuts, nut butters, seeds, avocado, and let's not forget the fats that are naturally occurring in whole foods. I recommend enjoying these added fats as part of a meal and not as a snack. If you set out to eat your daily ration of nuts, you may eat way more than you should. Instead, add nuts or seeds to your morning oatmeal, or your lunchtime salad. I could eat a cup of mashed avocado, but I'll happily eat much less when it is mixed with beans, grains, and salsa. I can get the fat I need without mindlessly eating too much.

Don't I Need Oil to Cook

If you eat a healthy, plant-based diet and still consume oil, you are doing better than most people I know. However, if you have heart disease, diabetes, or if you need to lose weight, I encourage you to give oil, even healthy oils, the boot, and see if it makes a difference. I discuss replacing oils in the chapter *Cooking for Health*.

Dairy & Eggs

I often joke that dairy is evil because it causes painful inflammation in my joints. While vegans do not consume animal products, including dairy and eggs, vegetarians may. I have read conflicting advice from plant-based experts. Most do not believe dairy and eggs belong in a healthy diet, but some of the doctors maintain that small amounts of dairy and eggs are permitted. There are factors that come into play here: first, health conditions which could be made worse by eating dairy or eggs; and second, ethical concerns. My husband and I chose not to consume dairy at all, but we occasionally ate organic, free-range eggs until we discovered that our son had egg allergies.

What About Fake Cheese

While I'm not a fan of fake dairy products, many people enjoy faux cheese, which can be made out of nutritional yeast or nuts. Since we are nut-free to accommodate our son's allergies, we usually stick to nutritional yeast. Faux cheese sauce can be used in recipes like mac & cheese, nacho cheese, or other casserole-like dishes.

Faux Milk

We use rice milk for most of our dairy needs. We enjoy the taste of almond milk and coconut milk as well. Hemp milk is a nutritious choice, especially for children. Soy milk is another option. If you need a replacement for buttermilk, mix one tablespoon of vinegar into one cup plant milk and allow it to set for about 10 minutes (this works best with soy milk).

Yogurt

There are many non-dairy yogurts available. They are typically more expensive than their dairy counterparts, but every bit as delicious. We've used soy, coconut, and almond milk yogurts in place of dairy for parfaits, fruit dips, and smoothie recipes. Plant-based yogurt (that is not flavored or sweetened) sometimes tastes a bit like sour cream.

Chapter Eight

But What About… A Few Frequently Asked Questions

There are a few questions that I get asked over and over again. I'm hoping to address them here, but some of the answers may not be black and white. The mission of this book is to equip you to eat healthier, not necessarily to persuade you to make changes. There are many books and websites available that can answer all of these questions from a medical perspective; I'll mention them in the resources section. Please speak with a qualified medical professional if you experience unpleasant symptoms or medical problems.

Whole Foods

Foods that are naturally unprocessed or minimally processed are considered whole foods. Some examples include fruits, veggies, beans, and grains. Whole kernel corn would be considered a whole food, while corn chips would not. Rolled oats are a whole food, but most oat-based ready-to-eat cereals are not. Food that has a long shelf life is typically highly processed and not a whole food.

I Feel Horrible, Maybe This Isn't for Me

If you eat the Standard American Diet, there is a good chance you will go through a bit of a detox when you clean up your diet and begin to eat healthier. Much of the food we eat is highly addictive and full of chemicals designed to keep us eating it. Almost everyone I know who has adopted a whole food, plant-based diet has gone through three days to two weeks of detoxing due to consuming fast food, caffeinated drinks, and loads of sugar, oil, and salt. Symptoms include headache, fatigue, brain fog, acne, or digestive issues such as gas, bloating, diarrhea, or constipation.

Your symptoms, if any, will depend on your diet prior to switching to a plant-based diet and what you choose to eat after.

Most often I hear from those eliminating caffeine that they have headaches and feel fatigue for about three days. When the detox symptoms last longer it is sometimes associated with food intolerances or allergies.

No matter the cause, these uncomfortable symptoms should subside soon, and you will probably find yourself feeling better than ever.

How Will I Get Enough Protein

Contrary to what you may have heard, plants contain protein. In fact, they contain enough protein to meet all your needs. As long as you eat enough calories, you should be getting enough protein.

Several years ago, fitness and nutrition experts perpetuated the idea that certain foods had to be combined for you to get a complete protein—containing all nine amino acids—or it wouldn't be beneficial. I remember a personal trainer giving me the same lecture. Newer research negates that theory, but many people still cling to it. If you eat a healthy variety of plants, you should be able to get all of the protein you need.

Supplements

The plant-based community is divided over the use of nutritional supplements. The experts I most closely follow contend supplements are not necessary as all nutrients can be received through a healthy diet. Other experts feel loads of supplements are needed. Both groups agree that people consuming a plant-based diet should supplement with vitamin B-12.

I take a different approach. I don't think people should take supplements unless they have a deficiency or medical issue that requires them. I have B-12 supplements, but I don't take them regularly. We drink rice milk and eat nutritional yeast; both are fortified with B-12. I take it occasionally if I feel it's needed. My most recent blood work showed excellent B-12 levels.

I encourage you to have a full blood workup completed by your doctor to become aware of any deficiencies. I attempt to make dietary changes instead of taking supplements, but I will supplement when necessary.

Often those beginning a plant-based diet will believe misinformation about nutrients and take unnecessary supplements. Some people may have underlying health issues that will require supplements, like iron, but that doesn't mean it's required for everyone.

Nutritional Yeast

Not to be confused with baker's yeast, nutritional yeast is a deactivated yeast, meaning it will not make bread rise. It is rich in B-12 and other nutrients that give food a cheesy or nutty flavor. I use nutritional yeast to make a faux cheese sauce and in my dry veggie broth mix. It tastes great in soups and sauces, or sprinkled on popcorn or baked potatoes.

Chapter Nine

Finding the Best Approach for You

What Kind of Person Are You

There are different kinds of people out there. Some people are jump-in-the-deep-end-even-though-it's-freezing kind of people, whereas others are wade-in-little-by-little-acclimating-as-you-go type of people. I get that and it's OK. Recognizing the kind of person you are (and the kind of people in your family) will be a tremendous help as you *transition* to a plant-based lifestyle. I say transition because, even if you cannonball into the deep end, there is a big learning curve. I have people whom I coach that think they jumped in and are doing great, but they don't realize their floaty sprang a leak.

Slow but Steady

Some people do better starting slow: using a systematic (planned) approach that makes gradual changes. To these people, I recommend removing ALL dairy first. You may experience withdrawal symptoms and feel horrible at first, it happens to a lot of people. Do not replace dairy with fake dairy-like products, you won't be doing yourself any favors. Once dairy is out of your system for two weeks, most people no longer crave dairy products. Tough it out, it is totally worth it.

Second, eliminate as much processed food as possible. The less processed foods you eat, the healthier your diet is. If you can't make it yourself, it shouldn't take up a lot of your food supply. Two of my exceptions are bread and tortillas. I choose to buy healthier options, but they are still processed foods.

Third, eliminate or reduce meat consumption to two to three ounces, two to three times per week. When my husband and I began our transition, we switched from conventionally-raised meat to organic free-range or grass-fed meat. We would buy it, bring it home, and immediately cut it into very small serving sizes and put it in the freezer. Eventually, we no longer bought meat at the store, but would occasionally have it when we went out to eat; now I choose not to eat meat at all. This was a slow progression; the first stage in our meat reduction went on for months. The second stage of eating meat only when we ate out went on for the better part of a year. At first it was once a week, then gradually once a month, and now it has been many months since I've had any meat.

Fourth, eliminate oil. "But, but…" No buts. Oil is not a health food. It is a concentrated source of fat without any nutrients. Olive oil, coconut oil, it doesn't matter, you don't need it.

All In

If you are ready to jump on in, take all of the steps in the above section and make today Day One. You can do it! It isn't near as hard or intimidating as you may think. Dairy, processed food, meat, oil: just toss them all.

Chapter Ten

Recipes

The following recipes are all reader favorites. They have been tested and approved time and time again. I'm sure your family will love them as well.

Crock Pot Mexican Rice and Bean Casserole

Ingredients

- 1 cup uncooked brown rice
- 3 cups water
- 1 (8 oz.) can tomato sauce
- 1 tsp. salt (optional)
- 1 tsp. onion powder
- 1 tsp. chili powder
- 1/2 tsp. garlic powder
- 1/2 tsp. cumin
- 2 cups cooked beans OR 1 can beans, drained (I use pinto and black beans.)
- 1 cup corn (optional)

Directions

Pour all of the ingredients into your slow cooker and stir gently. Cook on high for four hours or low for six to eight hours.

Enchilada Soup

Ingredients

- 6 cups veggie broth
- 1 diced onion
- 3 cups cooked beans (I use pinto and black beans)
- 1 cup diced tomatoes OR 1 can diced tomatoes
- 1 (8 oz.) can tomato sauce
- 2 cloves garlic OR 1 tsp. garlic powder
- 1 diced bell pepper
- 1 sliced jalapeno
- 2 cups cooked rice
- 1 cup corn OR 1 can corn, drained
- 1 small can diced green chilies
- 1 tbsp. chili powder
- 1/2 tsp. cumin
- salt to taste
- pepper to taste
- nutritional yeast (optional)
- tortilla chips

Directions

Bring veggie broth to a boil in a large pot. Add onions, cooked beans, diced tomatoes, bell peppers, jalapenos, corn, and rice. Give it a nice stir, then add tomato sauce and let simmer. Allow the soup to cook until onions are translucent and flavors have had a chance to meld. Add the remaining seasonings—chili powder, cumin, salt, pepper—then simmer for as little as a few minutes up to an hour.

Quinoa-Lentil Tacos

Ingredients

- 2 cups cooked quinoa
- 2 cups cooked lentils (brown or green)
- 1 1/2 tsp. garlic powder
- 1 1/2 tsp. onion powder
- 1 1/2 tsp. chili powder
- 1 tsp. cumin
- 4 oz. tomato sauce
- salt to taste
- pepper to taste
- crushed red pepper (optional, more spice)

Directions

If quinoa and lentils are cold, heat them in the microwave or on stove until warm. Mix all ingredients together in a large mixing bowl.

Notes

This is perfect for taco or burrito filling, but my favorite is on a taco salad.

Mexican Rice

Ingredients

- 1 cup brown rice (long or short grain)
- 2 1/2 cups water
- 6 oz. tomato sauce
- 1 tsp. salt (optional)
- 1/2 tsp. garlic
- cilantro (optional)

Directions

Pour rice into a skillet on medium heat. (I like to toast the rice a bit before adding water, but if you are too impatient you can skip that part.) Then add water and tomato sauce. (If you buy an eight ounce can you can use all of it if you'd like.) Next, add the salt and garlic.

Stir everything well then put a lid on the pan (the rice will cook best with a lid on). The temperature can be turned down once it is boiling. Check the rice at about 30 minutes, but it may need to cook closer to 45 minutes. It is done when most of the liquid is absorbed and the rice is soft. Allow the rice to cool for a few minutes before eating. Cilantro can be added on top of the rice after it is done cooking. Just sprinkle fresh cilantro on top of the rice and place lid back on skillet for a few minutes.

Notes

Use this recipe as a side dish or mix in beans, salsa, and guacamole for a meal.

Slow Cooker Potato Soup

Ingredients

- 6 medium potatoes, washed and cut into bite-sized chunks (I left skin on)
- 4 cups water
- 2 sliced carrots
- 1 diced onion
- 1/2 tsp. garlic powder
- 1/8 cup nutritional yeast
- salt to taste
- pepper to taste

Directions

Place water and all of the veggies into a slow cooker and set it to low for about six hours, or high for four hours. Add garlic powder and nutritional yeast, then mash with a potato masher until creamy.

Notes

An immersion blender will also work for a creamier soup.

Recipe can be doubled or tripled.

Very Vegan Chili (Texas Style)

Ingredients

- 3 cans of beans OR about 6 cups of cooked beans, any variety
- 1 diced medium onion
- 1 can diced tomatoes OR about 3 diced tomatoes
- 1 diced jalapeno
- 1 (8 oz.) can tomato sauce
- 1/4 cup chili powder (start with less and add more to taste)
- 1 tsp. garlic powder
- 1 tsp. cumin
- 1 tsp. paprika
- salt
- pepper

Directions

Dump the beans, diced onion, tomatoes, peppers, and tomato sauce into a large sauce pan and cook until onions, peppers, and tomatoes are cooked. Add spices to suit your individual taste preferences (we like a lot more chili powder than most people). Cook until everything is done and any extra liquid has cooked out.

Notes

This recipe can be doubled. It also freezes well.

Basic Stir-Fry

Throw this together based on leftover veggies from other dishes during the week.

Ingredients

- carrots
- celery
- onion
- broccoli
- bell peppers
- any other veggies that need to be eaten
- cooked brown rice OR quinoa OR noodles

Directions

In a hot skillet, add carrots and any other veggies that are hard and need the longest time to cook. (You do not need oil. If the veggies start to stick, add a spoonful or two of water to your pan.) Keep stirring veggies.

Next, add onions and peppers, followed by broccoli and other fragile veggies that don't need much cooking time. Once all of the veggies are cooked, dump cooked rice, quinoa, or lo mien noodles into skillet and gently stir.

Cover for a few minutes until heated through.

Notes

Use soy sauce or Braggs Liquid Aminos, if desired.

Banana Bread

Ingredients

- 1 cup applesauce
- 1/2 cup turbinado sugar OR raw sugar (I've also used agave with a good result)
- 3 mashed extra-ripe bananas
- 1 tbsp. plant milk
- 1 tsp. vanilla
- 1 tsp. baking soda
- 1/4 tsp. salt
- 2 cups whole wheat pastry flour
- 1/2 cup vegan chocolate chips (optional)
- 1/2 cup nuts (optional)

Directions

Preheat oven to 350°. Grab a large mixing bowl and add applesauce and sugar. Mix with wooden or sturdy spoon. Add the mashed bananas, plant milk, and vanilla; mix well. Dump in baking soda, salt, and flour; mix again.

You can add the optional nuts and/or chocolate chips now.

Pour batter into a sprayed pan (I use a bunt pan for best results). Cook for 40 minutes until a tooth pick comes out clean. (Using a loaf pan will require a longer baking time.) Remove from pan once cool.

Blueberry Muffins

Ingredients

- 1 cup applesauce
- 1/2 cup turbinado sugar OR raw sugar (I've also used agave with a good result)
- 2 mashed extra-ripe bananas
- 1 tbsp. plant milk
- 1 tsp. vanilla
- 1 tsp. baking soda
- 1/4 tsp. salt
- 2 cups whole wheat pastry flour (regular whole wheat flour can also be used)
- 1 cup fresh or frozen blueberries
- 1/2 cup nuts (optional)

Directions

Preheat oven to 350°. Grab a large mixing bowl and add applesauce and sugar. Mix with wooden spoon. Add bananas, plant milk, and vanilla; mix well. Dump in the baking soda, salt, and flour; mix again.

Add optional nuts and gently fold in the blueberries. Pour the batter into a sprayed muffin pan and cook for 25 minutes until a tooth pick comes out clean. Remove muffins from the pan once cool.

Notes

These muffins are a perfect snack or as part of brunch.

Brownies (Gluten-Free)

Ingredients

- 1/4 cup unsweetened applesauce
- 2/3 cup cocoa powder
- 1/4 cup brown rice flour
- 1/4 cup sorghum flour
- 1/4 tsp. sea salt
- 1/4 tsp. baking powder
- 1/2 cup turbinado sugar
- 2/3 cup pureed cooked sweet potatoes
- 1 1/2 tsp. vanilla
- up to 1/2 cup plant milk, start with 1/4 cup
- 1/2 cup vegan chocolate chips (optional)

Directions

Preheat oven to 350° and lightly spray an 8×8 pan.

Put all of the ingredients, except chocolate chips, in a large mixing bowl. Stir until everything is mixed well, adding more plant milk if needed. Fold in chocolate chips, reserving a few spoonful's. Spread the batter smooth and sprinkle the reserved chocolate chips on top.

Bake for 35 to 40 minutes; toothpick will **not** come out clean.

Notes

Allow these brownies to cool before cutting, if at all possible. This recipe doubles wonderfully: just use a 9×15 pan.

Chocolate No-Bake Bites

Ingredients

- 2 tbsp. cocoa
- 2 tbsp. agave OR maple syrup
- 1 tsp. vanilla
- 1 banana
- 1/4 cup peanut butter (or other nut or seed butter)
- 1 cup oats (use gluten-free if needed)
- 1/4 cup vegan chocolate chips (optional)

Directions

Mix together cocoa, agave, and vanilla in a medium-sized mixing bowl. (This will take a little while to do, but it will come together.) Mash in banana and stir. Mix in peanut butter (you can add another 1/4 cup for a stronger PB taste). Stir in oats, 1/4 cup at a time. If your mixture looks too dry, don't use all the oats. Add in the chocolate chips, if desired.

Roll mixture into balls or flatten into cookie shapes. Place them in the freezer or refrigerator to harden.

Notes

I store these in the freezer and grab one or two out for an after-dinner treat. Makes about 17 bite-sized cookies.

Chapter Eleven

Resources

PlantBasedPharmacist.com is a website run by the plant-based pharmacist, Dr. Dustin Rudolph. He offers information about diet, supplements, and health conditions. His blog, PlantBasedPharmacist.com, is full of great articles that will help you distinguish fact from fiction.

NutritionFacts.org is written by Michael Greger, M.D., and brings you important nutrition research, articles, and videos.

Engine2Diet.com is led by Rip Esselstyn, a former firefighter and professional athlete. It is a great resource for those wanting to make the move toward a plant-based diet. Engine 2 has books, a blog, and answers to your plant-based questions.

HappyHerbivore.com is a website and blog written by Lindsey S. Nixon. She is also a bestselling cookbook author who creates delicious recipes using everyday ingredients.

Forks Over Knives is a documentary about the state of our country's health. It discusses how most of the degenerative disease we face can be reversed or cured with a whole food, plant-based diet. Find the documentary and more at www.forksoverknives.com.

Dr. McDougall is a long-time leader in the plant-based movement. He has books, cookbooks, and a line of food. For decades he has helped people through immersion programs and has a free online program (www.drmcdougall.com) for people wanting to learn more about plant-based living.

Dr. Barnard is the founder of the Physicians Committee for Responsible Medicine (PCRM). He is the author of many books and a leader in the plant-based movement. Find him online at www.pcrm.org/media/experts/neal-barnard.

Dr. Kahn practices integrative cardiology and has developed an aggressive yet holistic approach to heart disease prevention and reversal. You can find him at www.drjoelkahn.com.

Dr. Fuhrman uses the term *Nutritarian* to describe this way of eating. He allows some meat and dairy, but focuses on high-nutrient plant foods. Find him online at www.drfuhrman.com.

Dr. Esselstyn specializes in heart disease; he became frustrated treating disease while doing nothing to stop it. He leads the cardiovascular prevention and reversal program at The Cleveland Clinic Wellness Institute. Find him online at www.dresselstyn.com.

Dr. T. Colin Campbell is probably best known for *The China Study* and is the chairman of the T. Colin Campbell Center for Nutrition Studies, found online at nutritionstudies.org. He teaches a whole food, plant-based diet as a way to avoid and reverse cancer and other illnesses common to those eating a Standard American Diet.

About the Author

Holly Yzquierdo lives in sunny Arizona with her family. They have been eating a mostly plant-based diet since 2011. Her youngest son has multiple food allergies that make cooking an adventure. She teaches classes on cooking, meal planning, and transitioning to a plant-based diet.

Holly blogs at MyPlantBasedFamily.com where she creates delicious, allergy-friendly recipes, free weekly meal plans, and offers tips to help you live a plant-based lifestyle.

32359654R00035

Made in the USA
Middletown, DE
04 January 2019